# Yummy in their tummy. Dog treat recipes to make at home.

Printed in the United States of America.
First addition
Published by Createspace and Beverly.K

# Author:  Beverly.K

# DOG Treats, You and your Pets are GoInG To Love.

## Simple

Dog treat recipes to make at home.

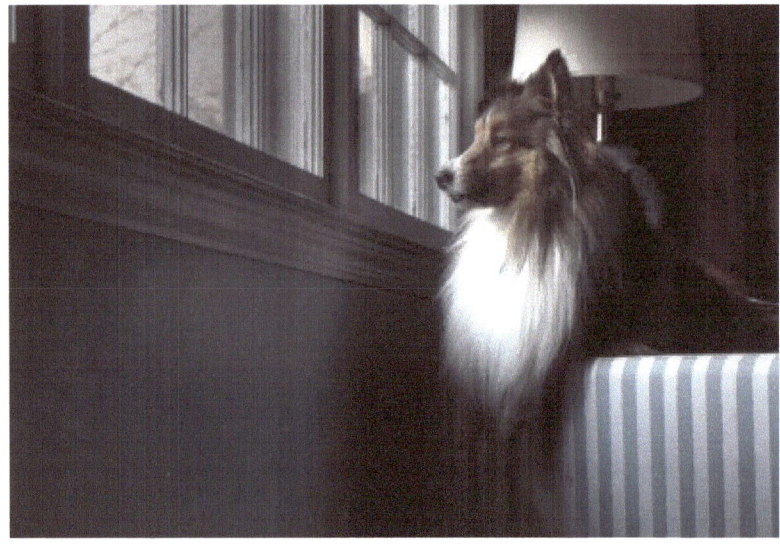

*Image courtesy of Ian Kahn / FreeDigitalPhotos.net*

# Things you will need to have on hand.

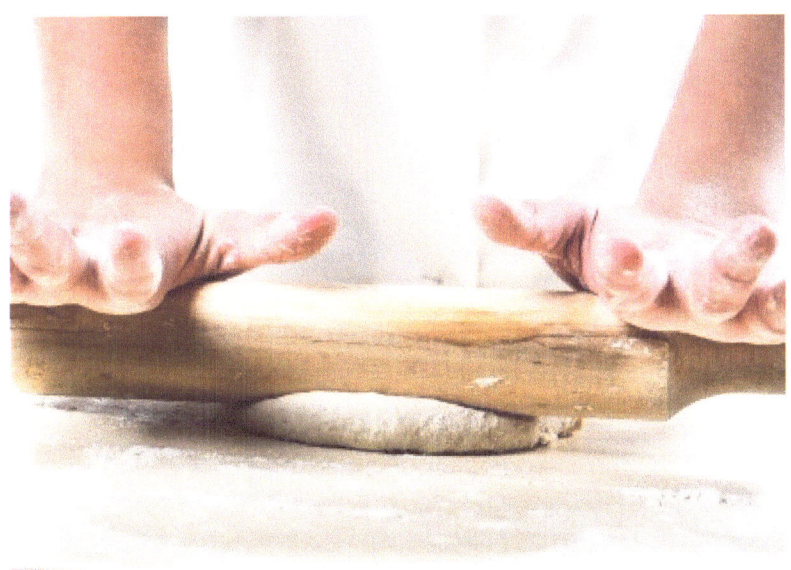

*Image courtesy of lemonade / FreeDigitalPhotos.net*

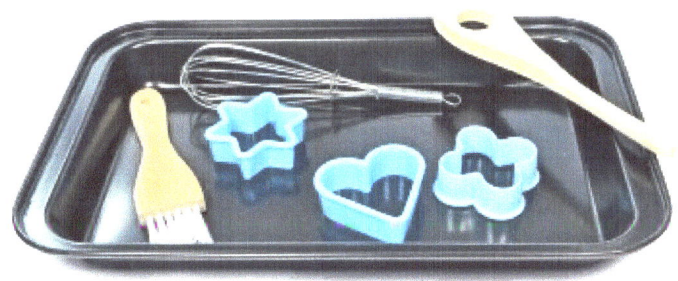

*Image courtesy of Grant Cochrane / FreeDigitalPhotos.net*

*Remember to always let the cookies cool down before giving them to your dog.*

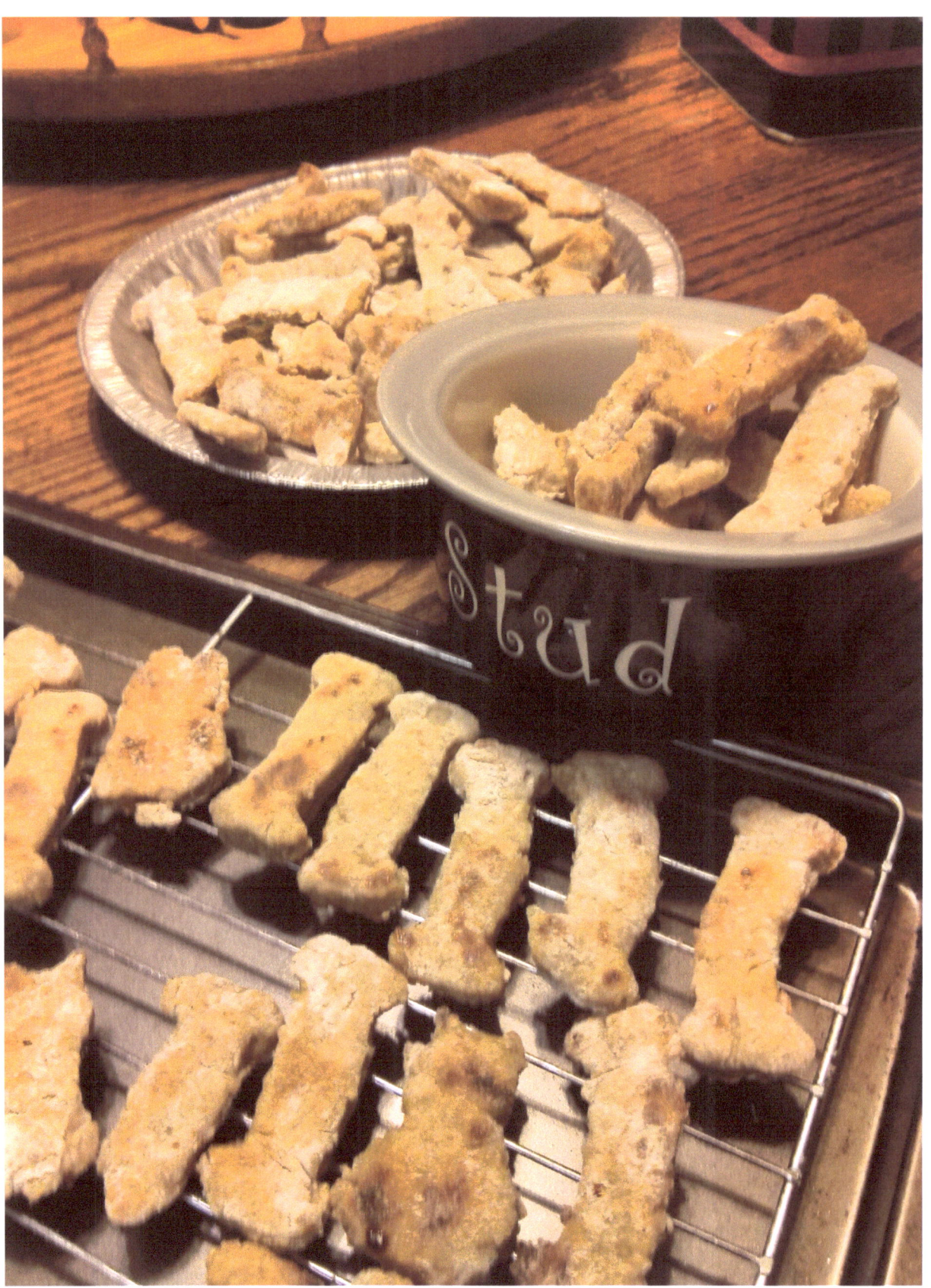

I began  working with animals 25 years ago. It seems like every animal is different when it comes to food.  Some can handle anything they put in their mouth.  Others may be allergic to certain thing.  Example wool, dog food, treats, toys, even bowls.

So learning what is good for your dog is not as easy as one may think.

This book is designed for  any dog  without allergies.  Read the recipes carefully to see which ingredients your pet may not be able to eat.

Some of you may have the doggy treat maker to cook them in.  If not just use a cookie sheet lined with parchment paper.

*If you have any questions or concerns about the ingredients used, please consult with your veterinarian.*

# PEANUT BUTTER TREATS

1/2 Cup peanut butter, creamy

1 Cup of water

1/4 Cup of honey

1 Cup flour

2 Cups rolled oats

2 Tbsp oil (olive oil)

Mix together in a medium bowl.
Knead dough into firm ball and roll out to 1/4 inch thick.
Cut into desired shapes and place on cookie tray. With parchment paper.
Time for the egg wash. This will make those biscuits nice, shiny, and smooth. Just beat an egg and brush it on the treats.
Oven temperature is 300
Cook till they brown about 40 minutes.

This batch made 70 bone shaped cookies.

Cool cookies on cooling rack.

Store treats into an airtight container or in the freezer.
Container is good for up to 2 weeks only.
Freezer is good for up to 3 months.

Do not feed your pet one right out of the freezer. Wait for it to thaw.

1/2 tsp of salt can be added to these treats to help extend the shelf life but, it is optional. Cinnamon is fine to use in recipes for dogs, however do not use a pumpkin spice blend or anything that could contain nutmeg. It is toxic to dogs and even in small amounts can make them sick.

# Peanut Butter Pumpkin

*1 cup pumpkin puree*

*2 eggs*

*1/2 cup oats*

*3 cups whole wheat flour*

*3 Tbsp of all smooth peanut butter*

*1/2 tsp cinnamon (optional)*


*Preheat oven to 350 degrees F.*

*In medium bowl, stir together the flour, oats, and cinnamon*

*In a separate large bowl, whisk together the eggs, pumpkin and peanut butter until combined. Stir wet ingredients into dry.*

*Pour onto a floured surface and roll dough out to 1/4 inch thick. Cut out using cookie cutter. The dough will be a little sticky, a dusting of flour for your hands and the rolling pin will help! Bake for 30 to 35 minutes until golden brown.*

*Place on cooling racks and let cool thoroughly. They will harden as they cool.*

Store treats into an airtight container or in the freezer.
Container is good for up to 2 weeks only.
Freezer is good for up to 3 months.

Do not feed your pet one right out of the freezer.  Wait for it to thaw.


1/2 tsp of salt can be added to these treats to help extend the shelf life but, it is optional.

Cinnamon is fine to use in recipes for dogs, however do not use a pumpkin spice blend or anything that could contain nutmeg. It is toxic to dogs and even in small amounts can make them sick.

# Sweet Potato Dog Biscuits

*1 cup of canned sweet potato or fresh sweet potato*

*1 3/4 cups whole wheat flour*

*1 egg (beaten)*

*Preheat oven to 350 degrees F.*

*Stir ingredients together in a large bowl until dough forms. Roll dough into small balls and place on a cookie sheet lined with parchment paper. Press dough down slightly so the biscuits are about about 1/4 inch thick. Bake until golden brown and let cool on a wire rack.*

Store treats into an airtight container or in the freezer.
Container is good for up to 2 weeks only.
Freezer is good for up to 3 months.

Do not feed your pet one right out of the freezer.  Wait for it to thaw.

1/2 tsp of salt can be added to these treats to help extend the shelf life but, it is optional. Cinnamon is fine to use in recipes for dogs, however do not use a pumpkin spice blend or anything that could contain nutmeg. It is toxic to dogs and even in small amounts can make them sick.

This was the very first batch I ever made.  I have improved much since then.
This is what they look like without the egg wash.

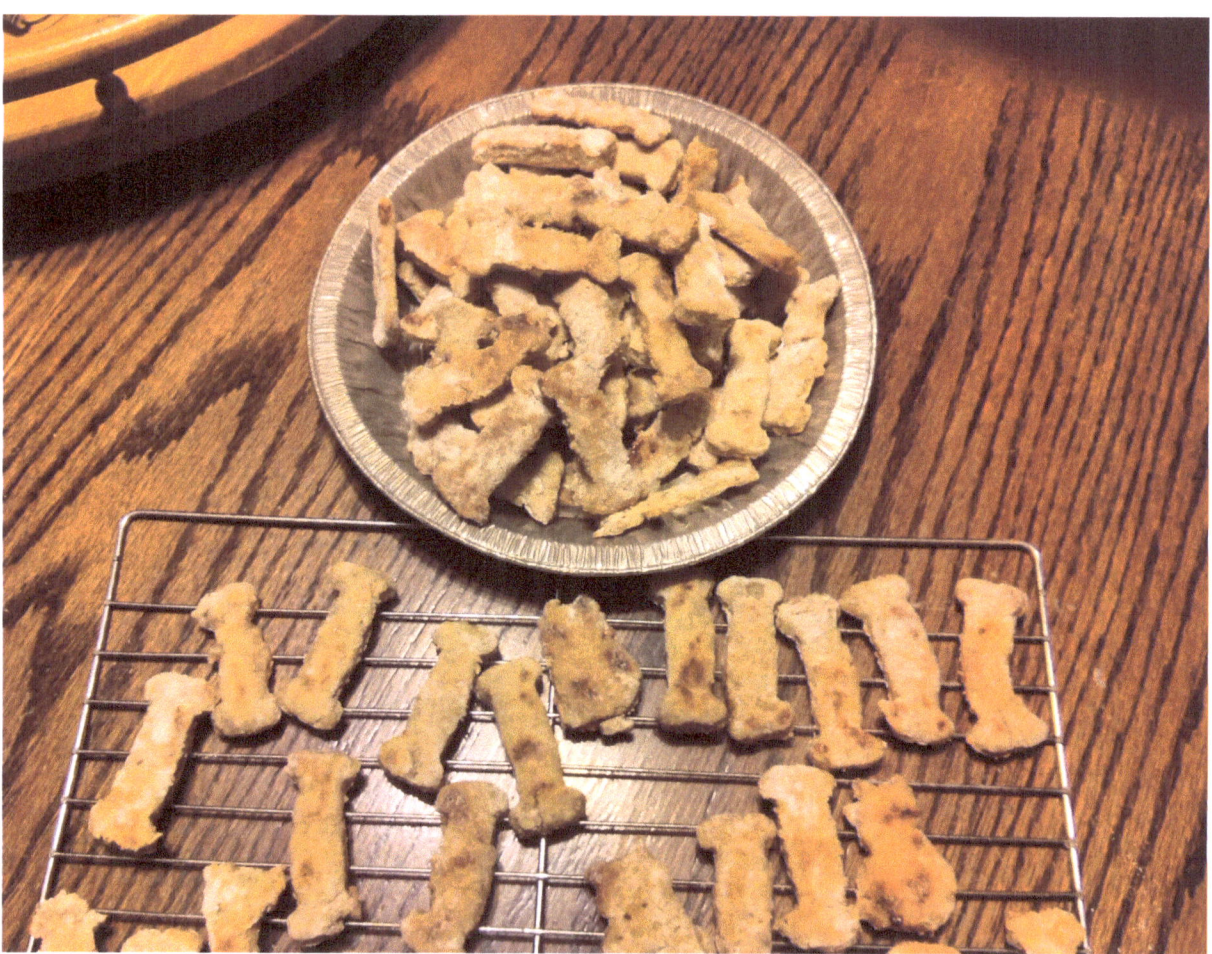

# Bacon and peanut butter

- 1 cup natural creamy peanut butter
- 3/4 cup nonfat milk
- 1 large egg (or 1/4 cup unsweetened applesauce)
- 2 cups whole wheat flour*
- 1 Tablespoon baking powder
- 1/3 cup oats (either whole-rolled or quick oats are fine)
- 2-3 strips bacon, chopped

Preheat oven to 325F degrees. Line two large baking sheets with parchment paper or silicone baking mats. Set aside.

In a large bowl, gently mix the peanut butter, milk, and egg together with a large spoon or spatula. Switch to a whisk to make sure no lumps remain. Add the flour and baking powder. You may need to turn the dough out onto the counter and use your hands to work in the flour. Mix in the oats and chopped bacon. The dough is extremely thick and heavy.

Using a rolling pin, roll the dough out into 1/4" thickness. Cut into shapes using cookie cutters or a knife. Arrange on the baking sheets. Bake for 18-20 minutes, or until very lightly browned on the bottom. Remove from the oven, and flip the treats to bake the other side for 10-12 more minutes.

Allow to cool completely before serving to your pup. Store at room temperature or in the refrigerator for up to 1 week. Treats freeze well, up to 2 months

Makes about 2 dozen treats.

# Apple Carrot Dog Treats

1 cup of whole wheat flour, brown rice flour, or gluten free flour

1 cup of grated carrots

1 tsp. baking powder

1 egg

1/2 cup unsweetened applesauce


Preheat oven 350 degrees F.  Till golden brown.

Mix ingredients together until dough forms. Roll dough into small balls and place on a cookie sheet lined with parchment paper. Press dough down slightly so the biscuits are about about 1/4 inch thick. Bake until golden brown and let cool on a wire rack.

***Makes about 2 dozen cookies*** Store treats into an airtight container or in the freezer. Container is good for up to 2 weeks only.  Refrigerate.Freezer is good for up to

3 months

# Oatmeal cookies

*2 cups rice 2 packages Reg. Flavor oatmeal (mixed w/milk)*
*1/4 cup molasses*
*1 cup carrots*
*1/3 cup spinach*
*1 1/4 cup flour*
*1/2 tbsp brown gravy mix*
*4 tbsp applesauce*
*1/2 tbsp vegetable oil*

*Preheat oven to 350 degrees Stir Ingredients, but adding flour gradually.*

*Drop on cookie sheet using tsp.*

*Bake 15-20 minutes or until golden brown. Makes around 2 dozen cookies.*

Store treats into an airtight container or in the freezer.
Container is good for up to 2 weeks only.  Refrigerate.
Freezer is good for up to 3 months.

# Skippy's treats

3 1/2 cup whole wheat flour

2 cup Quaker oats

1 cup milk

1/2 cup hot water

2 beef or chicken bouillon cubes

1/2 cup meat drippings

Dissolve bouillon cubes in hot water.
 Add milk and drippings and beat. In a separate bowl, mix flour and oatmeal. Pour liquid ingredients into dry ingredients and mix well. Press onto an ungreased cookie sheet and cut into shapes desired.

Bake at 300 for 1 hour. Turn off heat and leave in the oven to harden. Refrigerate after baking.

**Store treats into an airtight container or in the freezer.
Container is good for up to 2 weeks only.  Refrigerate.
Freezer is good for up to 3 months.**

## _This is Skippy_

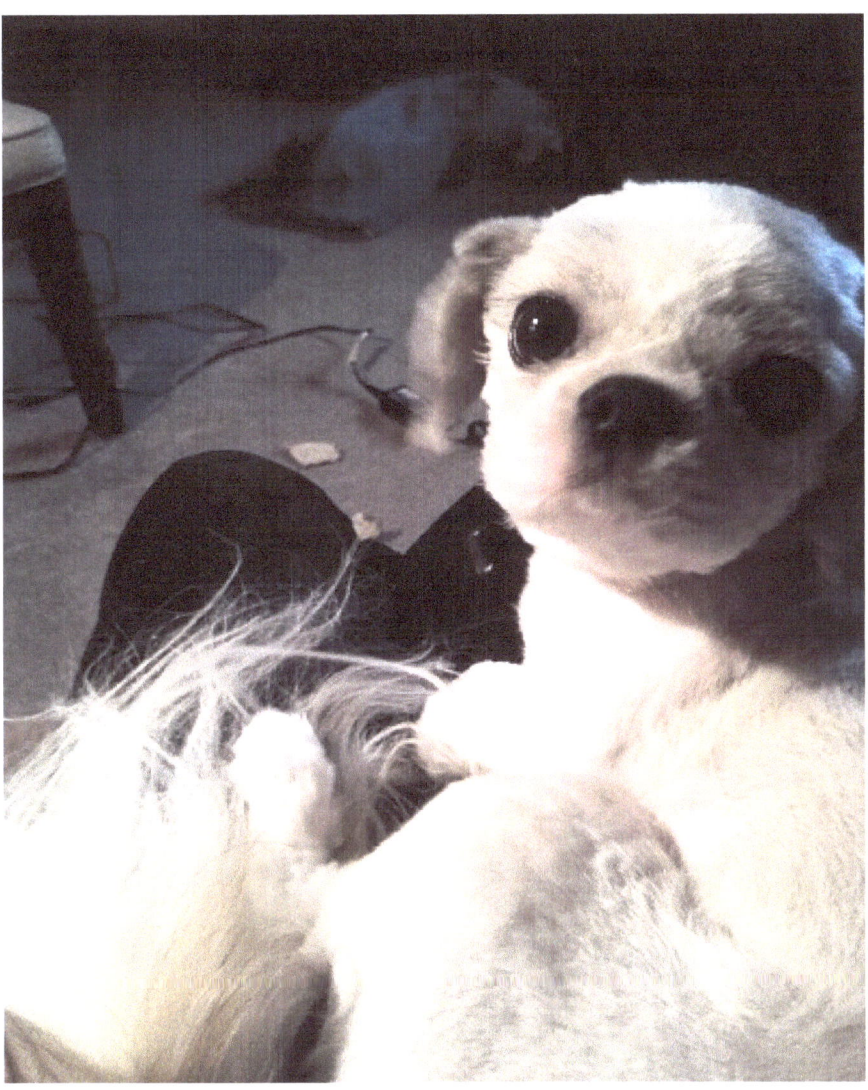

_Image courtesy of Beverly.K_

# Liver Treats

1 lb. beef liver
1 cup whole wheat flour
1 cup cornmeal
1 cup carrots shredded
2 eggs

Puree liver  in food processor. Add eggs, whole wheat flour and cornmeal. Make into shapes.

 Grease cookie sheet  or use parchment paper and pour mixture onto cookie sheet.

Bake in 350 oven for 20 minutes, flipping over halfway through baking. Cut into desired sized squares

**Store treats into an airtight container or in the freezer.**
**Container is good for up to 2 weeks only.  Refrigerate.**
**Freezer is good for up to 3 months.**

# Homemade Flax Seed Dog Biscuit Recipe

- 12 oz  whole wheat flour
- 12oz bread flour
- 2 oz  wheat germ
- 1 tsp salt
- 2 Tbsp brown sugar
- 3-4 Tsp Flax Seed (optional)
- 3 eggs
- 1 cup vegetable oil
- 3 oz  powdered dry milk
- 1 cup water

1. Combine wheat flour, bread flour, wheat germ, salt, and brown sugar, and flax seed in mixing bowl. Stir in eggs and vegetable oil.
2. Dissolve dry milk in water then incorporate the mixture.
3. Mix to form a very firm dough that is smooth and workable. Adjust by adding a little extra flour or water as required.
4. Cover the dough and set aside to relax for 15-20 min.
5. Roll the dough out to 1/2" (1.2cm) thick. Cut out biscuits using a bone-shaped cutter 3"x1.5" (7.5×3.7cm). Place the biscuits on sheet pans lined with baking paper.
6. Bake at 375°F (190°C) for approx. 40 minutes or until biscuits are brown and, more importantly, rock-hard. Let biscuits cool, then store in a covered container five to six feet off the flour. Use as needed to reward your four-legged friends.)
7. **Store treats into an airtight container or in the freezer.**
8. **Container is good for up to 2 weeks only.  Refrigerate.**
9. **Freezer is good for up to 3 months.**

Tip for cute cookie cutters.  Check out your closest dollar store.

# Banana  logs

**2 1/4 cups whole wheat flour**
**1/2 cup powdered milk -- nonfat**
**1 egg**
**1/3 cup banana -- ripe, mashed**
**1/4 cup vegetable oil**
**1 beef bouillon cube**
**1/2 cup water -- hot**
**1 tablespoon brown sugar**

**Mix all ingredients until well blended. Knead for 2 minutes on a floured surface.**

**Roll to 1/4 " thickness.  Bake for 30 minutes in a 300 degrees oven on ungreased cookie trays or cookie tray with parchment paper.**

**Shape into a Tootsie roll. There you go. You now have banana logs.**

Store treats into an airtight container or in the freezer.
Container is good for up to 2 weeks only.  Refrigerate.
Freezer is good for up to 3 months.

# Parmesan cheese treats

*2 1/3 cups flour -- all-purpose or whole wheat*
*1/4 cup olive oil*
*1/4 cup applesauce*
*1/2 cup grated cheese -- like parmesan*
*1 large egg*
*1/4 cup powdered milk -- non-fat*

*Combine all ingredients in a large bowl; mix well; Roll the dough out to size of a cookie sheet;*
*cut out your design*
*place on cookie sheet*

**Time for the egg wash. This will make those biscuits nice, shiny, and smooth. Just beat an egg and brush it on the treats.**

*Bake in a 350 degree oven.*
*Cook for 20 minutes or until golden brown.*

**Store treats into an airtight container or in the freezer.**
**Container is good for up to 2 weeks only.  Refrigerate.**
**Freezer is good for up to 3 months.**

# **Emmy's pies.**

12-16 ozs. raw liver
1 1/2 lbs. white flour
8 ozs. Quaker Oats
3 bouillon cubes, (meat or chicken flavored)
Approx. 1 cup water
2 eggs, beaten


Preheat oven to 350F.
 Grease 3 baking sheets or use parchment paper
 Chop the liver finely, by hand or in food processor.
Mix flour and oats, crumble in the bouillon cubes, add eggs and the chopped liver.
Add enough water to make a firm but slightly sticky dough. Spread evenly on the sheets about 1/2" thick.
Dip a small dog-biscuit cutter in flour before cutting out each portion.
 Remove uncut parts, use that for next pan. Spread out on another cookie sheet and repeat. Bake 1 hour or until golden brown.


Store treats into an airtight container or in the freezer.
Container is good for up to 2 weeks only.  Refrigerate.
Freezer is good for up to 3 months.

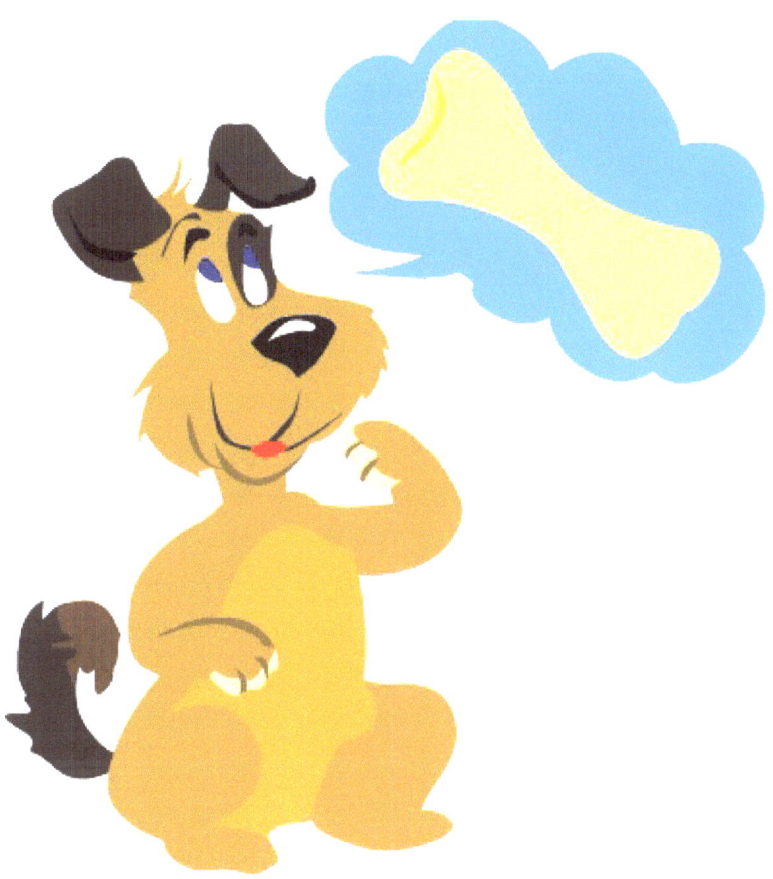

# Chicken Biscuits

1 1/2 cups shredded cooked chicken
1/2 cup low sodium chicken broth
1 tbsp butter
1 cup whole wheat flour
1/3 cup cornmeal or cream of wheat.

Combine chicken, broth and butter and blend well.
Add flour and cornmeal or cream of wheat.
Knead dough into a ball and roll out to 1/4 inch thick.

Cut out your design with cookie cutter.

**Time for the egg wash. This will make those biscuits nice, shiny, and smooth. Just beat an egg and brush it on the treats.**

Cook at 325 till golden brown.

Remove from oven and let cool down on cookie rack.

Store treats into an airtight container or in the freezer.
Container is good for up to 2 weeks only.  Refrigerate.
Freezer is good for up to 3 months.

# *Veggie munchies*

3 tsp fresh parsley minced.
1/4 cup carrots, shredded
1/4 cup shredded cheddar cheese
2 tbsp olive oil
2 and   3/4 cup flour
2 tbsp bran
2 tsp baking powder
1/2 tsp flaxseed (optional)
1/2 cup water

mix together in medium bowl
knead dough into a firm ball
roll out to a 1/4 inch thick
cut into desired shapes
place on cookie sheet with parchment paper.

Time for the egg wash. This will make those biscuits nice, shiny, and smooth. Just beat an egg and brush it on the treats.

Oven 300 degrees.
Cook till golden brown.

 Store treats into an airtight container or in the freezer.
Container is good for up to 2 weeks only.  Refrigerate.
Freezer is good for up to 3 months.

# Bacon  paws

6 slices of bacon ( cooked and crumbles )
4 eggs beaten
1/8 cup of oil
1 cup water
1/2 cup powdered milk
2 cups flour
2 1/2 cups wheat germ


Mix together in a medium bowl.
Shape into balls
Use the bottom of a coffee cup to flatten each ball to 1/4 inch thick.
make a paw print on each one using your thumb for the big part of
a dogs pad and your finger to make the toes.

Time for the egg wash. This will make those biscuits nice, shiny, and smooth. Just beat
an egg and brush it on the treats.

Cook at 300 degrees until they are golden brown.
depending on the size you made.

Store treats into an airtight container or in the freezer.
Container is good for up to 2 weeks only.  Refrigerate.
Freezer is good for up to 3 months.

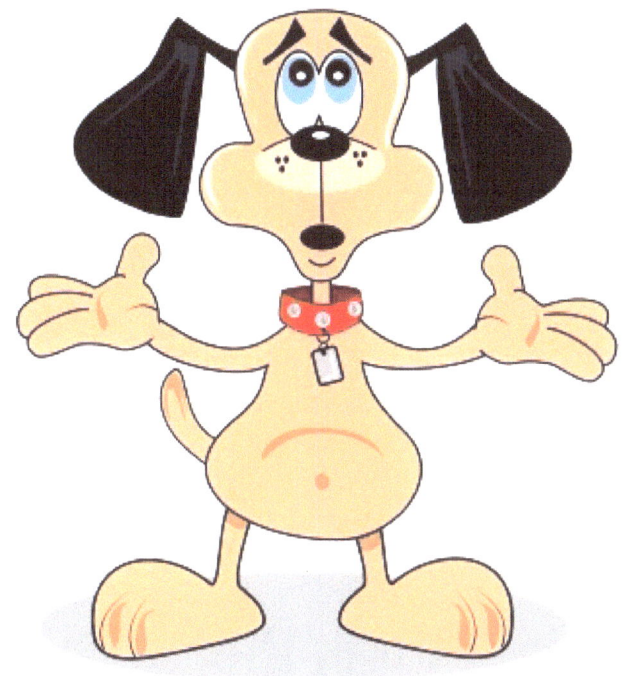

## Dangerous Foods for Dogs

Who can resist those big brown eyes and cute doggie grin? Can a little reward from the table really hurt your dog? Well, that depends on what it is and what's in it. A chip with guacamole can cause your dog some real problems. In fact, there's a lot of people food your dog should never eat. And, it's not just because of weight. Some foods are downright dangerous for dogs -- and some of these common foods may surprise you.

## Avocado

No matter how good you think the guacamole is, you shouldn't give it to your dog. Avocados contain a substance called persin. It's harmless for humans who aren't allergic. But large amounts might be toxic to dogs. If you happen to be growing avocados at home, keep your dog away from the plants. Persin is in the leaves, seed, and bark, as well as in the fruit.

# Alcohol

Beer, liquor, wine, foods containing alcohol -- none of it's good for your dog. That's because alcohol has the same effect on a dog's liver and brain that it has on humans. But it takes far less to do its damage. Just a little can cause vomiting, diarrhea, central nervous system depression, problems with coordination, difficulty breathing, coma, even death. And the smaller the dog, the greater the effect.

# Onions and Garlic

Onions and garlic in all forms -- powdered, raw, cooked, or dehydrated -- can destroy a dog's red blood cells, leading to anemia. That can happen even with the onion powder found in some baby food. An occasional small dose is probably OK. But just eating a large quantity once or eating smaller amounts regularly can cause poisoning. Symptoms of anemia include weakness, vomiting, little interest in food, dullness, and breathlessness.

## Coffee, Tea, and Other Caffeine

Caffeine in large enough quantities can be fatal for a dog. And, there is no antidote. Symptoms of caffeine poisoning include restlessness, rapid breathing, heart palpitations, muscle tremors, fits, and bleeding. In addition to tea and coffee - including beans and grounds -- caffeine can be found in cocoa, chocolate, colas, and stimulant drinks such as Red Bull. It's also in some cold medicines and pain killers.

## Grapes and Raisins

Grapes and raisins have often been used as treats for dogs. But it's not a good idea. Although it isn't clear why, grapes and raisins can cause kidney failure in dogs. And just a small amount can make a dog ill. Repeated vomiting is an early sign. Within a day, the dog will become lethargic and depressed. The best prevention is to keep grapes and raisins off counters and other places your dog can reach.

# Milk and Other Dairy Products

On a hot day, it may be tempting to share your ice cream cone with your dog. But if your dog could, it would thank you for not doing so. Milk and milk-based products can cause diarrhea and other digestive upset as well as set up food allergies (which often manifest as itchiness).

# Macadamia Nuts

Dogs should not eat macadamia nuts or foods containing macadamia nuts because they can be fatal. As few as six raw or roasted macadamia nuts can make a dog ill. Symptoms of poisoning include muscle tremors, weakness or paralysis of the hindquarters, vomiting, elevated body temperature, and rapid heart rate. Eating chocolate with the nuts will make symptoms worse, possibly leading to death.

## Candy and Gum

Candy, gum, toothpaste, baked goods, and some diet foods are sweetened with xylitol. Xylitol can cause an increase in the insulin circulating through your dog's body. That can cause your dog's blood sugar to drop and can also cause liver failure. Initial symptoms include vomiting, lethargy, and loss of coordination. Eventually, the dog may have seizures. Liver failure can occur within just a few days.

## Chocolate

Most people know that chocolate is bad for dogs. The toxic agent in chocolate is theobromine. It's in all kinds of chocolate, even white chocolate. The most dangerous kinds, though, are dark chocolate, chocolate mulch, and unsweetened baking chocolate. Eating chocolate, even just licking the icing bowl, can cause a dog to vomit, have diarrhea, and be excessively thirsty. It can also cause abnormal heart rhythm, tremors, seizures, and death.

# Fat Trimmings and Bones

Table scraps often contain meat fat that a human didn't eat and bones. Both are dangerous for dogs. Fat trimmed from meat, both cooked and uncooked, can cause pancreatitis in dogs. And, although it seems natural to give a dog a bone, a dog can choke on it. Bones can also splinter and cause an obstruction or lacerations of your dog's digestive system. It's best to just forget about the doggie bag.

# Persimmons, Peaches, and Plums

The problem with these fruits is the seeds or pits. The seeds from persimmons can cause inflammation of the small intestine in dogs. They can also cause intestinal obstruction. Obstruction is also a possibility if a dog eats the pit from a peach or plum. Plus, peach and plum pits contain cyanide, which is poisonous to both humans and dogs. The difference is humans know not to eat them. Dogs don't.

○

## Raw Eggs

There are two problems with giving your dog raw eggs. The first is the possibility of food poisoning from bacteria like Salmonella or E. coli. The second is that an enzyme in raw eggs interferes with the absorption of a particular B vitamin. This can cause skin problems as well as problems with your dog's coat if raw eggs are fed for a long time

## Raw Meat and Fish

Raw meat and raw fish, like raw eggs, can contain bacteria that causes food poisoning. In addition, certain kinds of fish such as salmon, trout, shad, or sturgeon can contain a parasite that causes "fish disease" or "salmon poisoning disease." If not treated, the disease can be fatal within two weeks. The first signs of illness are vomiting, fever, and big lymph nodes. Thoroughly cooking the fish will kill the parasite and protect your dog

# Salt

It's not a good idea to share salty foods like chips or pretzels with your dog. Eating too much salt can cause excessive thirst and urination and lead to sodium ion poisoning. Symptoms of too much salt include vomiting, diarrhea, depression, tremors, elevated body temperature, and seizures. It may even cause death

## Sugary Foods and Drinks

Too much sugar can do the same thing to dogs that it does to humans. It can lead to obesity, dental problems, and possibly the onset of diabetes

## Yeast Dough

Before it's baked, bread dough needs to rise. And, that's exactly what it would do in your dog's stomach if your dog ate it. As it swells inside, the dough can stretch the dog's abdomen and cause severe pain. In addition, when the yeast ferments the dough to make it rise, it produces alcohol that can lead to alcohol poisoning

## Your Medicine

Reaction to a drug commonly prescribed for humans is the most common cause of poisoning in dogs. Just as you would do for your children, keep all medicines out of your dog's reach. And, never give your dog any over-the-counter medicine unless told to do so by your vet. Ingredients such as acetaminophen or ibuprofen are common in pain relievers and cold medicine. And, they can be deadly for your dog

## Kitchen Pantry: No Dogs Allowed

Many other items commonly found on kitchen shelves can harm your dog. For instance, baking powder and baking soda are both highly toxic. So are nutmeg and other spices. Keeping food items high enough to be out of your dog's reach and keeping pantry doors closed will help protect your dog from serious food-related illness

## If Your Dog Eats What It Shouldn't

tDogs explore with their mouth. And, no matter how cautious you are, it's possible your dog can find and swallow what it shouldn't. It's a smart idea to always keep the number of your local vet, the closest emergency clinic, and the ASPCA Animal Poison Control Centre

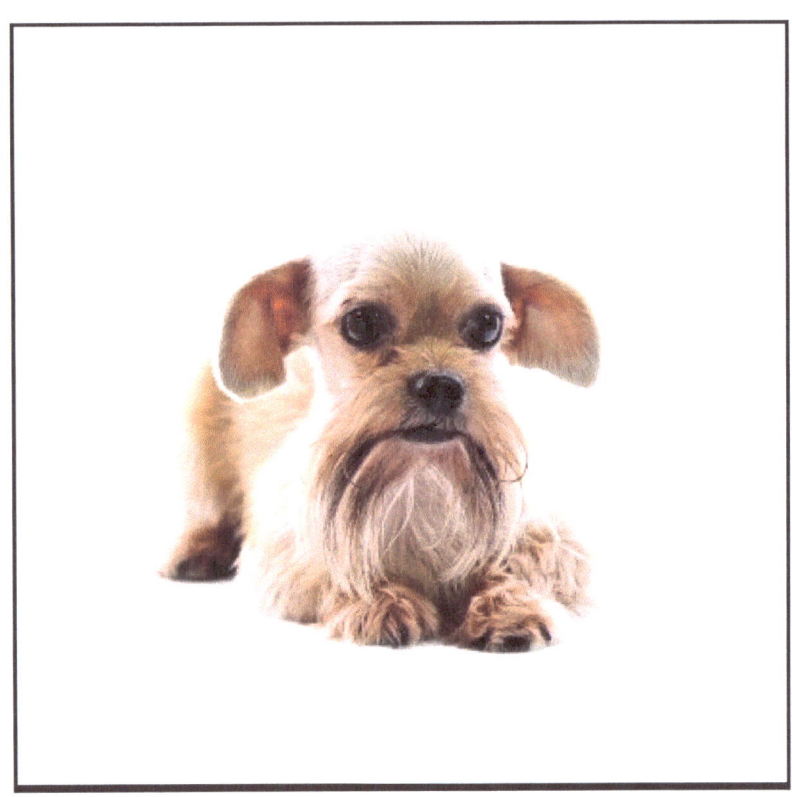

# What Dogs Can Eat

You can ensure your dog has a healthy, well-balanced diet by asking your vet to recommend a quality dog food. A well-designed dog food gives your pet all the nutrients it needs for an active and healthy life. But that doesn't mean you can't sometimes give your dog human food as a special treat -- as long as portions are limited, and the foods are cooked, pure, and not fatty or heavily seasoned. See the next few slides for some tasty suggestions. But if you're looking to human food as a meal replacement, talk to your vet about amounts and frequency.

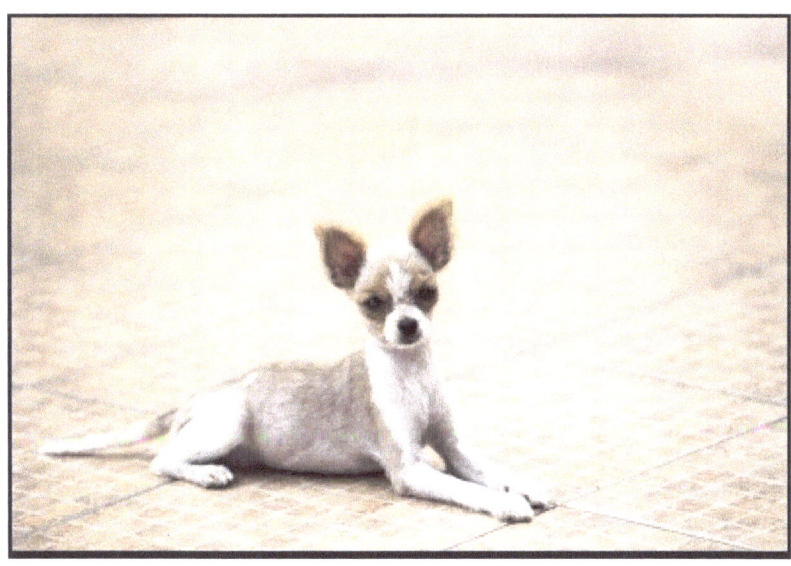

*Image courtesy of khunaspix / FreeDigitalPhotos.net*

## Safe: Lean Meats

Most dogs are fine eating lean cuts of meat that have been thoroughly cooked. Be sure to remove all visible fat -- including the skin on poultry. Also be sure that there are no bones in the meat before you give it to your dog.

## Safe: Some Fresh Fruits

Slices of apples, oranges, bananas, and watermelon make tasty treats for your dog. Be sure to remove any seeds first, though. Seeds, stems, and leaves can cause serious problems.

## Safe: Some Vegetables

Your dog can have a healthy snack of carrot sticks, green beans, cucumber slices, or zucchini slices. Even a plain baked potato is OK. Be sure, though, not to let your dog eat any raw potatoes or any potato plants it might have access to in your garden.

## Safe: Cooked White Rice and Pasta

Dogs may enjoy plain white rice or pasta after it's cooked. And, a serving of plain white rice with some boiled chicken can sometimes provide welcome relief from gastrointestinal upset.

# Dont  forget to cool down the cookies before you feet them to your pet.

*Image courtesy of Bill Perry / FreeDigitalPhotos.net*

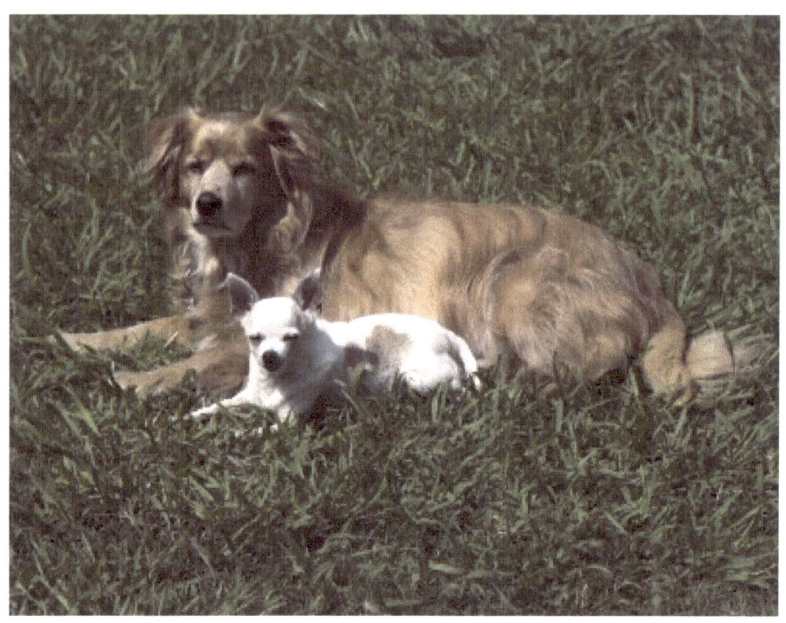

Thank you for checking out my book. If you have any recipes you would like to share with me, I would be more than happy to try them and maybe put them in a new book with your permission to use your recipe and acknowledge you in the book.

What I am looking for is more treats and dog food recipes. If you would be willing to share your cat recipe with me, I will also check them out and may use them in the next book with your permission of course. Please send me a review of this book if you can along with recipes you would like to share to my mail box. I will then send you a permission form for your recipe and a picture of your pet who will also be mentioned in the book. If you are just interested in a notice of any other books that are published by me I will let you know first before the public If you send your email address.

Please email me at www.bmkillaire@gmail.com

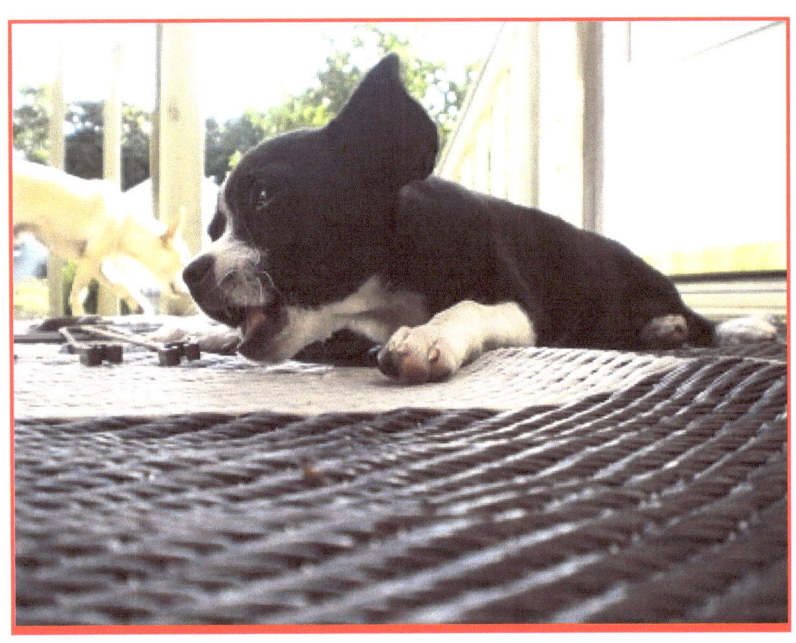

**Photo permission of B.M.Killaire**